The Patient's Journey

Mapping, analysing and improving healthcare processes

Sarah W. Fraser

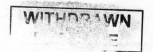

Kingsham

First published in 2002
by Kingsham Press

Oldbury Complex
Marsh Lane
Easthampnett
Chichester, West Sussex
PO18 OJW
United Kingdom

© 2002, Sarah W. Fraser

Typeset in AGaramond

Printed and bound by
MPG Books
Bodmin
Cornwall
United Kingdom

ISBN : 1-904235-09-3

All rights reserved. No part of this book may be reprinted or reproduced or utilised in any form or by any electronic, mechanical, or other means, now known or later invented, including photocopying and recording, or in any information storage or retrieval system, without the prior permission in writing from the publishers.

British Library Cataloging in Publication Data
A catalogue record of this book is available from the British Library

Fraser, Sarah.

About the author

Sarah W. Fraser is a Visiting Professor at the University of Middlesex and an Independent Consultant. She has had a number of operational and management roles in both the private and public sector including Esso/Exxon and the NHS. Her area of expertise and consultancy at national and international level focuses on improving performance through developing leadership and organisational capability. She uses quality improvement methodologies as well as insights from systems thinking and the complexity sciences.

Contents

Introduction

Patients experience health care services in many different ways. They access statutory and non-statutory, public and private organisations in pursuit of advice, diagnosis, treatment and support.

The patient's journey is a complex and often frustrating one, involving them in deciding where to go, how to get there, coping with delays and doubling back. It is often a journey into the unknown, with uncertainties at every junction. For someone who is not well, this journey can be stressful and unproductive.

One of the fundamental starting points to improving health care services is to focus on these journeys that patients experience. By making the current situation explicit to all those involved in supplying health services through mapping what actually happens and then helping them analyse what is going on, you can discover ways to improve the patient's experience.

This guide takes you through the activities of mapping, analysing and then improving patient processes. It is a practical guide and if you are interested in some of the theory, then the annotated bibliography will provide you with a reading list.

Each topic is dealt with quite briefly and most of the chapters are stand-alone. With the exception of the section on mapping where the sequence of reading is important, every other part of the guide can be accessed and used as stand-alone hints, tips and explanations of what to do.

If you've never mapped a process before

The first section on "getting started" is designed to help you through the first steps of mapping a process, from finding a team to help you, through to agreeing the specific patient process, the format and level of detail you'll work to.

Ways to map processes are covered in "mapping"; you'll find it much easier to learn about mapping if you actually have a process in mind as you use this guide. You might find it best to leave the sections on "analysing" and "taking action" until you've mapped your first process. The section on facilitating is worth reading early on.

If you've experienced mapping and want to learn more

You can skip the "getting started" section though you might find it useful to refresh yourself on the practicalities of agreeing the format and level of detail of the process you have decided to map, analyse and improve.

The focus for you will be the "analysing", "taking action" and "facilitating" chapters. There are many new and updated ideas, hints and tips that you may find useful to extend your knowledge of how to get the most out of patient process mapping.

This workbook does not set out to be a definitive how-to guide. The experience of the author is that there are many different ways to improve processes and it is this richness, diversity and creativity that is fundamental to the change process. You'll find this guide prompts your thinking in a structured way. It is your answers, your thoughts and your experience that matters.

Chapter 1

What is mapping?

Gillian, the clinical nurse specialist (CNS) in the endoscopy suite has just returned from a meeting with the audit department. One of the issues that the recent departmental audit raised was the lack of a common route through the department for patients undergoing an upper gastro-intestinal endoscopy. She felt the reason for this was that they were adjusting their way of working to suit each patient so that the best possible service was provided. However, the audit manager explained that the amount of variability meant there was a lot of wasted time and in fact good service and clinical outcomes might not be as reliable as the patient should be able to expect. He showed the way the audit facilitator had tracked some patients through the procedure. There seemed to be at least four different ways to have the endoscopy done and there didn't seem to be any logic as to why they were different.

The audit department had also carried out some patient interviews and Gillian read though them. She was struck by how many referred to their experiences as a journey. They mentioned going step by step along a pathway, with various decisions and turns. Looking at the process map, she suddenly saw the link between the way in which the patient moved around the endoscopy suite and the comment about their journeys. The map was a representation of what actually happens and for the first time she was able to see that the procedures they carried out in the endoscopy suite were in fact only part of the whole of the patient's experience of the hospital.

A **map** is a representation of features; it highlights the main characteristics of the area showing how they are connected and where the choices are, so a different direction can be taken. It provides the reader with as wide a view as possible, so they can see the best way forward, where the short cuts are and where they might be delayed. Whilst it seems obvious, it's important to remember that the map is not the reality – the map of London is not London itself. Similarly the map of the patient's journey is not the journey itself.

Key features of a map

- Sense of the whole, or at least the wider picture
- Shows the routes
- Identifies choices and decision points (junctions)
- Provides opportunity to plan progress
- Shows connections and short cuts

Mapping is the process by which you represent the activities and steps experienced by the patient. This is a diagnostic and analytical process of discovering what actually happens. You can then use this information to find ways to improve how the patient experiences the care you deliver. Another name for mapping is **flowcharting**; *charting the flow* of people, information, materials etc. Mapping a process, therefore, is creating a visual representation of the sequence of steps and activities that the patient experiences.

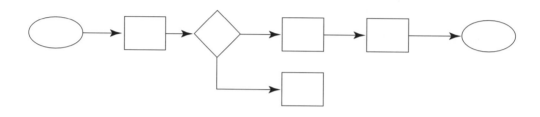

Chapter 2
What is a process?

Gillian was concerned about how she could sort some of the problems raised by the departmental audit. It wasn't clear to her what a "process" meant. Is this the same as the clinical procedures they do? The audit facilitator assured her that some of this was the same. However, the big difference was that the process was something seen from the **patient's point of view** and not any one member of the clinical or managerial team. This meant it covered all the different groups in the organisation that contribute to the upper GI process.

After a quick review she worked out that at least seven different departments contributed to a simple upper GI process; general medicines, pathology, sterile supplies, stores, human resources, accounting, maintenance. There were probably more.

The audit facilitator pointed out that there were very many *inputs* to a process; manpower, equipment, materials, procedures and methods. All of this goes into the *process* whereby a patient experiences an upper GI endoscopy.

Gillian asked how it is decided all these inputs go into the process. The facilitator answered by explaining that purpose was important – what are we trying to achieve. This indicates the *output* that is the result of the process. In most cases for the upper GI procedure, the output is a diagnostic report and an indication of whether treatment is required or not.

A process transforms inputs into outputs ...

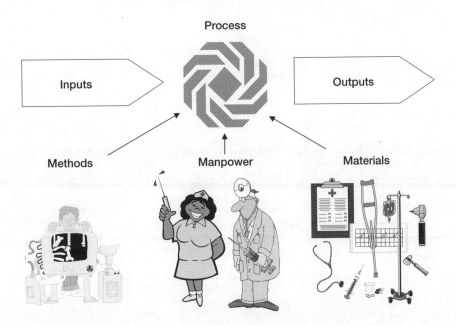

Process

Inputs

Outputs

Methods   Manpower   Materials

Every process has at least one **output**. This is the main operational purpose of the process. This can be a diagnostic report (from an upper GI endoscopy), a set of new skills (acquired through the process of training), a set of results (from the pathology laboratory) etc.

The **process** is the means by which the output is delivered. It is characterised by the way it uses a variety of **inputs**, such as materials and equipment, different people and their abilities as well as formal and informal methods and procedures. The process mixes up all the inputs and produces an output.

Chapter 3
Why map?

The departmental team meeting had not gone well. The audit department's review of the endoscopy suite created a lot of dissension and discussion. There were many different points of view about the patient's journey. It was obvious the explanatory diagrams the audit department used to explain the amount of variability and duplication were creating upset and confusion.

Gillian decided they would need to do their own process map, perhaps in a more specific and detailed way. She thought it was the one way that the complexity, confusion and duplication could be made explicit to everyone in the department.

The audit facilitator thought this would be a good idea, especially if members of the department were involved in the mapping process. He also offered to benchmark the map against the endoscopy unit in a neighbouring hospital, so they could see how well their performance compared.

There were obviously a lot of changes needed to the services provided by the endoscopy team and Gillian thought that mapping would be a way to not only find out what is currently going on, but also to identify where they can make improvements. Depending on the result, the map could even be used as a training tool for new members of the team.

Mapping helps teams to identify the actual flow or sequence of events that the patient experiences. Why is this useful?

✓ Helps the team to see the whole picture of the patient's journey and not just the parts in which they are involved.
✓ Enables the identification of the duplication of effort and wasted time and resources (both staff and patient or carer)
✓ Identifies where the real problems are, where further investigation and analysis may be required
✓ Shows the complexity of the patient's journey, from their perspective (often the clinical and administrative procedures seem very simple when viewed from the point of view of the member of staff)
✓ Highlights issues and activities that cross different functions in the organisation
✓ Provides a baseline against which changes can be measured and future performance compared

One of the most important reasons for carrying out a mapping process is to identify what happens now, and how patients and staff feel about the process. It is essential that you enter into a mapping exercise with the aim of identifying the *current situation*, not mapping out what you or the rest of your team think should happen.

Section A

Getting started

Preparation is key. Facilitators and project managers who have rushed into mapping will all tell you that they regret not organising the exercise properly.

What can go wrong right at the start?

- Not enough people who are involved in the process, participating in the mapping exercise
- Forgetting to include those who are not in your department yet who are still involved in the patient process
- Lack of agreement to provide required information
- What is excluded from the process is not clear
- The start and end points are uncertain
- Start by getting into too much detail without prioritising using a high-level overview map first

This section focuses on these problem and takes you through:

- ✓ How to select the team to support you in the mapping exercise
- ✓ What issues you need to cover to gain agreement from your colleagues for their participation in the process
- ✓ The importance of selecting and defining the patient process that you have chosen to analyse
- ✓ The options for the format and level of detail of your map

The activities in this section will involve you in quite a lot of discussion with your colleagues. The amount of time it takes to define your choice of process will depend on many factors. This could all be completed in an afternoon meeting, or you may find that it takes longer to fine-tune the details and gain commitment from others to participate in this work.

Chapter 4

Select a team

Gillian wondered who should be on the team to help her carry out the mapping task. She certainly wasn't going to do it on her own. She met with the diabetes CNS, Adrian, to see what advice he could offer her.

He explained that his mapping project had not gone very well, for many different reasons. One of them was because he did the map entirely on his own. Apart from the exercise being a very stressful and demand one on his time, he felt that this made it much more difficult to share with others once it had been completed. He explained there were many disagreements about the validity of the map and even when they agree to make some changes, his colleagues never really seemed to believe there really was a need to make improvements.

Gillian asked him what he would do if he were starting all over again. He suggested she involve a multidisciplinary team, and this needs to include at least one of the consultants. Getting patients involved in some way would also be useful. Perhaps by asking them to check the results, or even giving them notebooks and asking them to record their experiences.

What about facilitation and the technical aspects of mapping? Adrian thought Gillian would be quite able to facilitate the process herself. To some extent it was no more challenging than the regular monthly clinical governance meeting. As to the technicalities, well, they won't take long to learn.

Process mapping is a team activity and one best carried out by members of the team who are eventually going to be involved in making changes to the way they work. It is tempting to call in a project manager or another outsider to do the mapping. This may mean the task gets completed a little more quickly, however, it also means the learning that is the result of the mapping process, then resides with someone who is not part of the process being mapped. This learning is very important. The process of mapping enables improvement as it starts to create the tension for change. Besides – mapping is fun, so why let someone else do it!

The mapping team should include:

❑ Five to eight people
❑ As many different disciplines and roles as possible. This includes both clinical and administrative roles.
❑ A patient or a carer; as a minimum you should engage with patient and carers after you have completed your map
❑ One or two of the team members may come from outside your immediate department as they may be involved with the process e.g. pathology laboratory, stores, maintenance etc.

❑ If you feel unsure, then ask one of the audit department or process improvement facilitators to joint the team to help you while you learn how to map a process

There is no specific experience required to help map a process. The most important requirement is that the mapping team members are mostly the people who actually deliver the services and activities that the map will cover.

Chapter 5

Agree to map

Gillian felt she had a long way to go with her colleagues in the endoscopy department before they would be able to start mapping. The diabetes CNS, Adrian, has warned her that it was vital to get agreement from her co-workers before she started. He had run into problems where some of the doctors, nurses and secretaries had not wanted to give his team the information they needed. Sometimes this was a definite "no", other times it was more about their sudden "unavailability" and unwillingness to be involved in the process. Adrian felt all this was exacerbated by the fact the mapping exercise had been instigated by someone from outside their department and it was seen as a management performance type arrangement rather than an improvement related one.

At the next departmental meeting, Gillian argued to have a 15-minute slot to discuss the mapping exercise and to get commitment from others to be either active participants or at least willing information sharers.

Agenda issues for the departmental team meeting

❑ Drivers for change (what are all the reasons why we are under pressure and need to come up with improvements)
❑ The advantages of mapping the process
❑ Shortlist of processes to map (which ones, from the patient's perspective, appear to give the most problems)
❑ Who needs to participate in the mapping team?
❑ Mapping plan (who will do what with whom and by when)
❑ Access to data (implications for collecting data from team members)
❑ Commitment to the process (agreement to go ahead, with provisos if necessary)
❑ Next steps (when to meet, what more needs to be done before we start)

There is no set way to gain commitment to the mapping exercise. You may decide to use a meeting, or you may spend time with each one of your colleagues, convincing them of the benefits and opportunities of a process map as a means of finding ways to resolve some of the improvement challenges facing you. A good test of whether you have commitment to the exercise is to check for:

✓ Volunteers to participate
✓ Recognition of the need to improve
✓ Agreement that new solutions need to be found
✓ No one is actually trying to stop you carrying out the exercise!

Chapter 6

Select the process

Gillian had reached an agreement for the upper GI process to be mapped. This was the culmination of much debate that started with mapping the process for anyone entering the department. She decided this was so broad that they wouldn't get enough of the right details to help them improve their performance and the patient's experience.

The audit facilitator has made the job a little easier by the preliminary work that had been done. This had highlighted the upper GI process as one needing improvement. Also, the process improvement facilitator had suggested they work on a process that was fairly routine and one that had a high throughput of patients. This was not easy to achieve. Many of Gillian's co-workers wanted to work on the processes that gave them the most problems, such as urgent inpatient bronchoscopies. However, there were not many of these patients and the procedure tended to be performed on an irregular basis. Gillian eventually convinced her colleagues that it was better to make an improvement on a larger base of patients, such as the upper GI process.

"Focus on the patient's perspective"

Finding the process

Some processes are fairly easy to recognise, such as the one for upper GI endoscopies. Others are a lot more complex, usually because they are hidden in the midst of a large number of constantly interacting activities – a messy system. For example, many diagnostic processes, such as that for lung cancer, are difficult to identify, as they seem to belong to so many 'other' processes. The trick is to look at what is going on from the patient's perspective; what is the process they experience?

Choosing the process using patient groupings

Early business process re-engineering work at Lucas Industries in the UK identified three types of customer or product processes – *runners*, *strangers* and *specials*. These apply equally well to patient processes.

	Runners	Strangers	Specials
Volume	High (80%)	Low (16%)	Very low (4%)
Throughput speed	Fast	Slow	Very slow
Predictability	High	Moderate	Low
Standardisation	High	Moderate	Very low
Pre-scheduled	Most	Some	None

You should choose a process that is from the "runners" category. It may feel overwhelming to start with what looks like a large amount of patients and a significant process, however, just a small change here could have a large overall impact. For example, would you rather save 10 minutes per patient per week for a total of 100 patients ($10 \times 100 = 1000$ mins per week, which is 52000 mins per year, which is 867 hours in a year, or nearly 100 working days), or 30 minutes per patient per week for a total of 4 patients (104 hours or 12 working days)? Specials are just that – special. They will always need extra time and the advantage of optimising the runners is you can then find more time for those who need it most.

Chapter 7

Define the process

Gillian soon discovered that defining what is part of the upper GI process wasn't as simple as it sounded. Each of the four consultants managed their referrals for upper GI procedures in a different way. Also, they handled some upper GI procedures at another nearby community hospital. Should these be included?

One of the secretaries met with Gillian and volunteered to join the mapping team. She wanted the process map to start from the time the general practitioner (GP) send her the referral letter. She felt this was where the problems started. Gillian wasn't sure about this. Her preference was to start the process when the patients arrived in the clinic at the hospital.

Even more debate happened over when the process map should end; when the procedure was complete, when the report was generated, when the letter was sent back to the GP, when the patient was formally discharged with no need for further treatment – when?

The beginning... and the end...

Every process map needs to have an agreed start point for the process and an end point. This does not mean it is the beginning and end of the patient's process, just that it is the beginning and end of the map.

Processes hide in messy systems

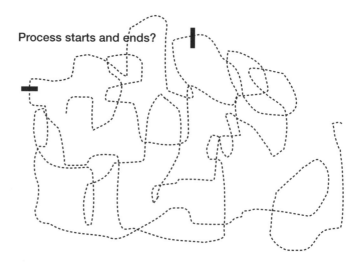

Process starts and ends?

Why are beginnings and endings important?

...to manage anxiety:
Mapping a patient's journey is part of the process of change. Most people are uncomfortable with change and they can get very anxious about anything that may mean they have to work in different ways. If it is not clear what and who is included or excluded from the process map, many people who may not actually be affected will still be concerned and may get stressed.

...to manage the mapping exercise:
Once you start the mapping process many interesting and apparently relevant issues that you will want to include will sidetrack you. As a result, the map will grow and grow until it no longer reflects the original purpose and aims you set out at the start of the exercise.

Before you start mapping your process, you need to gather some more information and decide on the following:

1	Name of your process	Give it a name that reflects the patient's perspective and also describes the process to be mapped.
2	Process owner	The person who is ultimately responsible for the process. This may be a team, in which case the team leader is the process owner.
3	Process output	Describe the output of your process – what is created; what is the end result? For example, is it perhaps a report or a sample?
4	Who is involved in delivering the process	List all the roles and departments who are involved in the process. You need to ensure they are either represented on the mapping team, invited to meetings or are receiving updates on your progress.
5	Who cares about the process *(but not directly involved in delivering it)*	Some people require you to do certain things in the process, even though they are not involved. For example, the audit department may be interested in the way you follow up results from their last audit.
6	What is excluded from the mapping exercise	Any special areas that will not be included. For example, activities that take place in the neighbouring community hospital.
7	The start	State clearly the start point for the mapping exercise. For example, when the GP makes a decision to refer a patient to the hospital for an upper GI endoscopy.
8	The ending	State clearly where the map intends to end. For example, when the report is posted to the GP.

It is highly recommended that you document the above and circulate it to all the mapping team members as well as all those who are directly or indirectly involved with the patient process. You may find you have to make some changes after you start the mapping process, but at least you will have the foundations for discussion and an excellent base from which to benefit from the mapping exercise.

Chapter 8

Agree level of detail

Adrian met Gillian over lunch and told some horrific tales of what he called "death by mapping". She was intrigued. Apparently on the diabetes project they started by mapping out every single activity and task along the process. They went down to details such as "patient arrived", "patient waited in queue at reception", "patient handed over appointment letter", "letter checked against the appointment list", "Patient waited in waiting room" etc.

Obviously this is what the patient experienced, but Adrian explained they spent so much time capturing all this detail that the map became unmanageable. They also ended up mapping in detail parts of the process that were not a problem, which was a waste of time and effort.

Gillian thought she would do her map differently. She decided to start by sketching out a map at a very high level, to get just an overview of the key activities and steps of the process. Then, after some analysis and discussion with the team, she would decide where they needed to carry out more mapping in more detail.

Mapping and analysing is not a linear process. The product of your mapping exercise is predominantly the learning and knowledge you gain about your process. You need to plan for carrying out a number of mapping exercises that start by capturing an overview and then move into more and more detail.

High-level overview map

This is a flowchart that contains the 6–9 key activities in the process. Use this to check your start and end points are appropriate. It is also a good way for the mapping team to get to know one another. You might find that some of the team want to get into more detail. Ask them to wait for the next step where their skills will be very useful. If you have defined your process well, a high-level map should take you no longer than a couple of hours to complete.

High-level example

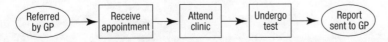

Next levels

After you've completed your overview, you can then choose which part you feel would be the most appropriate to do in more detail. For example, if the reporting process appears complex, with duplication and delays, then you may wish to capture what happens in more detail.

"Start with an overview, then map in every increasing detail."

Chapter 9
Choose a format

Gillian stopped by Adrian's office to see what his process maps looked like. From a beginners perspective they looked a real mess! She had expected them to be neatly typed flowcharts rolled up in bundles. Instead she found lots of flipcharts with Post-it™ notes and arrows going in all directions. It took her a while to work out which direction the patient was flowing in the diagrams.

Adrian explained that he used three different formats for doing the maps. He wished he'd stuck mostly with one, but it ended up that all three were useful at some time in the project. He declared the most important thing was to decide which format you were going to use before you started each new map. Otherwise you end up in a muddle and spend more time sticking paper together than you do on understanding the process.

There are three basic formats. It is best to start with either a **horizontal** or **vertical** format (whichever one you prefer) and move on to the **top down** version when you are more skilled at mapping.

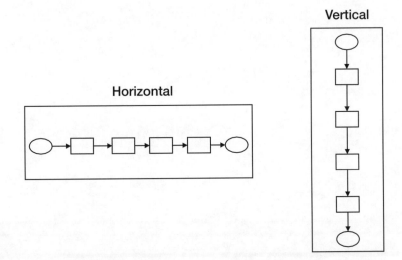

The **top down format** (see diagram on the next page) is very useful for more detailed mapping and can help speed up the analysis process as it shows the different activities and the people and roles involved in each.

Top down

	GP	GP Secretary	Clinic Secretary	Patient
Decides to refer				
Prepares and sends letter to clinic				
Receives letter via post room				
Organises appointment				
Sends patient letter giving date				
Sends GP copy of letter				
Letter arrives with GP secretary				
GP receives information about the appointment				

Section B

Mapping

The best way to learn about mapping a patient process is to do one! There is no perfect way to develop a visual representation of the patient's journey and there are no rules that the product, your map, must meet in order to be worthwhile. Any effort to make the current process explicit is a helpful one.

Whilst the focus of this section is on how to produce a process map, it's worth remembering that the action of mapping, the teamwork and discussions that happen, are as important as the map itself. Facilitating the mapping process is not without its challenges (see section E for more information).

Before you start mapping you need to have:

- ❑ Formed a mapping team (chapter 4)
- ❑ Defined your process (chapter 7)
- ❑ Agreed whether you will start with a high level map or a more detailed one (chapter 8)
- ❑ Chosen a format (chapter 9)
- ❑ Set aside at least two hours for the first exercise (chapter 11)
- ❑ Found a place to meet, where you have enough table space to use sheets of flip chart paper
- ❑ Sufficient materials to hand; flip chart paper, Post-it™ notes (different colours and shapes are helpful), marker pens

There are four steps to creating your process map:

1. Identify the key activities or tasks
2. Put these into sequence; the order in which they currently happen

3. Identify the key decisions that influence the route the patient takes
4. Draw the connections between the activities and the decisions

This section describes each of the four steps. It starts with an explanation of the symbols and shapes used in the diagramming process. Whilst these shapes are useful tools for the design of your map, the map has equal value if you choose to ignore these or even design your own.

Chapter 10

Symbols and shapes

Gillian noticed that Adrian's maps had some shapes. He explained that there were many different shapes and symbols that could be used for flowcharting. In fact a course he'd been on had gone through over fourteen of them! Adrian also explained that he used Post-it™ notes a lot as they could easily be moved around the flip chart paper. When he as too lazy to draw the different shapes he used different colours of Post-it™ notes.

Whilst she was interested in the ways in which the shapes could be used, Gillian was more concerned with why it was necessary to use them. Adrian explained that it helped you see what was going on in the map – at a glance. He pointed out that the diamond shapes always showed decision points. As decisions are good opportunities for change, it's worth being able to spot them quickly. Likewise, he felt using the circle shapes for beginning and ending the map was also helpful.

There are four symbols and shapes that you will need to be familiar with to diagram your patient process:

Rectangle ▢	**Activities, tasks, steps in the process** This is the most commonly used shape. You write in it a short description of the activity. This should include a verb (doing word) as well as the role of the person doing it and the subject to which it refers e.g. GP decides to refer patient, patient attends clinic.
Diamond ◇	**Decisions** This poses a question that needs an answer – yes or no. With the question in it. Use arrows to flow out of the points of the diamond to show alternative responses:
Circle ○	**Start and end steps** You should have at least two of these in your map. You can also use this symbol to show where the patient process moves to another department or phase, not included in your mapping exercise.
Arrow →	**To connect each of the activities, decisions or start and end points** Everything should be connected with an arrow.

Options

❑ Rectangles or squares for activities? There's no difference so use either.

❑ Use Post-it™ notes for the rectangular activities/tasks shape
❑ Use different coloured Post-it™ notes to represent the different shapes
❑ A diamond shape is just a square turned 45 degrees; use square Post-it™ notes, preferably in a different colour to the ones used for activities/tasks

Chapter 11

Identify activities

The endoscopy department had finally agreed Gillian's notes on the definition of the patient processes they were going to be working on. She had most of the mapping team in place and was pleased to see that the information systems department had agreed to send someone. Not only would this person probably have useful experience on flowcharting, she would also be key when it came to resolving some of the long delays in communications between primary care and the hospital – the post took far too long and Gillian hoped that an email based solution would be found.

Gillian had read some notes about how to map and seen the ones Adrian's team produced for the diabetes project. Although the symbols and shapes looked a little confusing at first she reckoned that most of the map would be the activities, some decisions interspersed, and a circle at each end, connect it all with arrows and hey presto! – There would be the map. It looked like the most time consuming and valuable place to start would be identifying the activities.

The mapping team decided to start by doing a high level map of the top 6–9 steps in the Upper GI process. This meant they had to find the key activities, steps or phases of the patient's process.

Before you go any further, check you have:

❑ Defined your process (chapter 7)
❑ Agreed whether you will do a high level map to start with, or go straight into more detail (chapter 8)
❑ Chosen a format; horizontal, vertical or top-down (chapter 9)

The skeleton of a map is the activities, steps or tasks that comprise the patient process. You need to identify and agree the key 6–9 activities (if you are doing a high level map, more if you are doing a more detailed one).

1. The **first activity** (written in a circle) is the starting point of the process that you should have already agreed (chapter 7)
2. The **last activity** (also written in a circle) is the activity that ends your process. This is often related to the output. For example, "consultant produces report".
3. The **activities in between** are all written in rectangles:

High level mapping

- *Focus on the current situation,* what actually happens now, not what you would like to happen (you'll get to that later – chapter 27)
- Brainstorm onto Post-it™ notes, one activity per note.
- If you get stuck, ask yourself "what happens next".
- Group these and see if you can find the common steps to help you simplify your map. *For example, "Post room delivers letter", "Secretary opens letter", "Secretary enters details onto computer" – could all be simplified, at a high level, into one activity "Secretary receives and deals with referral letter".*

More detailed mapping

- Spend more time brainstorming the activities onto Post-it™ notes. Make sure everyone in the team contributes, even if they think an activity happens in someone else's area.
- Aim to collect at least 50 activities. You can always summarise them later.

Fine-tuning your activities

The brainstorming process is a very creative one. You will end up with a mix of activities, decisions, delays, guesses and assumptions. The heat of the moment will have produced a mass of paper that may be difficult to read. It's important to involve the rest of the mapping team in this fine-tuning process.

a) Clarify the wording

Work through the notes and rewrite each one making sure you are phrasing the activity in a simple and clear way. You should try and use the name or role of the person, a verb and an object. *For example, "nurse preps patient", "consultant carries out procedure", "secretary types letter".*

b) Set aside decisions and other information that is not currently relevant

Chapter 13 covers decisions in more detail. At this stage you should weed out and save any activity that looks like it is a decision – it can be answered with the words yes or no. A decision is a point in the process where the patient could travel in different directions, depending on how the question is answered. *For example, "Is the referral urgent?" or "Is there sufficient time to complete the procedure?"*

c) Check the activities all refer to the current situation

Despite your best efforts you may find that ideas on how the process should work, not how it works now, will have crept into your map! If some of the activities are assumptions, then discuss with the team how you might verify whether they are true or not.

d) Check the activities fall within the agreed boundaries for the process map

Your process definition will have included the start and end points of your process, as well as what is excluded. Make sure the activities you have collected so far fit within these boundaries. If you find the team wants to add new areas to the map be very cautious. Sometimes it is necessary to change the boundaries, however, you will need to go back to the agreement stage of this exercise (chapters 5 to 9).

e) Carry out a final brainstorm or data capture process; check what's missing

The fine-tuning process always throws up a number of activities that no one remembered in the first pass of brainstorming. Allow enough time to capture these.

Don't be too concerned about the level of detail you have captured (whether it is enough or too much). Completing the first phase of your map will be an iterative process and you should be prepared to go round the loop of chapters 11 to 14 a few times before you've finalised your map.

Chapter 12

Sequence activities

The meeting to brainstorm and gather all the activities they could think of went very well. Perhaps too well. Although Gillian had planned to do only a high level map at this stage, she found they had gathered far more activities, in more detail, than she had expected. In just over an hour they collected over 100 steps in the patient process. They then spent nearly two hours fine-tuning and rewriting the steps so they were clear, simple and directly relevant to the patient process they had selected.

However, she felt very overwhelmed by all the detail and couldn't see how the team was ever going to reach the point where they had it all organised and pinned up on the wall. Adrian's advice was to take a day or so to reflect after the meeting, and then she could start to put the activities into the right order. It would be best if the mapping team did this, but she could make a start at it if she thought it would help.

"Sequencing – putting the activities in the order in which they happen"

Your map is of a patient process and the viewpoint for sequencing should be that of the patient.

The easiest way to organise your activities is to start by finding the high level steps. Set these down across the top of a piece of flip chart paper. Then put each one of the activities under these headings. Don't worry if one is repeated; you can fine-tune that detail later on.

For example:

Referral	Booking	Attend clinic	Report
GP decides to refer	Appointment date chosen by secretary	Patient attends clinic	Consultant enters test results into computer
Secretary types letter	Secretary writes letter to patient	Nurse completes admission process	Nurse prints out report
Letter posted to hospital	Patient receives appointment letter	Patient waits in waiting room	Secretary sends report to GP
Letter arrives with secretary		Patient undergoes test	

High level map

This should be a fairly straightforward process. Your sequence is simple as you have only a few activities in the map. The key is to find a way to summarise the steps that makes the most sense to your improvement activity.

Detailed map

You will need to check you have all the steps and there are none missing. Then make sure you have them organised by key step (as in the example above). At this stage you might decide you need to get even more detail for one step e.g. the booking process. If so, go back to "identify activities" and repeat the process.

You are now ready draw your high level map or to add decisions if you are doing a detailed version, after which you'll be able to make the connections and create your detailed map.

Chapter 13

Identify decision points

Gillian didn't see why decisions were needed as part of the map. Despite feeling overwhelmed with information only the week before, now that the team had organised and sequenced the activities she felt far more in control of the mapping process. In fact, it looked like they had a map already – only the arrows connecting the activities were missing. She thought that adding decision diamonds would make the map messy.

On Wednesday afternoon Gillian was in the upper GI clinic doing what she always did as a CNS; supporting her team, making sure the clinic ran smoothly, helping the consultants with the procedures and caring for patients. Mid way through the clinic it was obvious they were going to have at least three patients not attending. Gillian had to decide whether to end early (which was favourite with all the staff) or ring up some of tomorrow's patients who lived close to the hospital and see if they could come in at short notice.

All of a sudden she realised why the patient process map needed decisions. There were real choices that had to be made. Sometimes these were part of the regular scheduled process, like does the patient need to be seen this week or can they wait a couple of weeks, or they could be due to changes that happen on the spur of the moment, like sudden cancellations or no-shows.

Gillian resolved to get the mapping team together to look at the major decision points in their process. She also made some notes about finding ways to solve the no-show problem. She thought they could return to that when they analysed and improved the process.

"Adding decision diamonds to your map is done at the detailed level; high-level maps don't have decisions."

Why are decisions interesting?

❏ They make explicit the different people involved in the patient's journey and provide information about the roles they play
❏ Decisions are often factors in delaying or interrupting the smooth flow of the patient through the health care system
❏ They highlight duplication of effort e.g. each person in the process requesting personal information from patients before they are allowed to progress

How are they identified?

- Decisions happen between activities; identify the top 10 key activities and ask "who needs to decide what, so that this activity can take place?"

How are they phrased in the process map diamonds?

- They must end in a question mark
- They must be answered with either a "yes", or a "no"; *for example, "Does the patient need to be seen this week – yes/no", "Is the endoscopy equipment ready – yes/no".*
- Be clear and specific. If the question can't be phrased in a simple way, and it is an important one for the mapping process, then you may need to break it down into more detailed activities and minor decisions

How do the diamonds work?

They are junctions on your map. Each decision diamond splits the route into at least two different directions. A third direction is possible if you don't know the answer to the question and have to double back (a good thing to find as this is often a waste of resources and a delay in the patient's journey!).

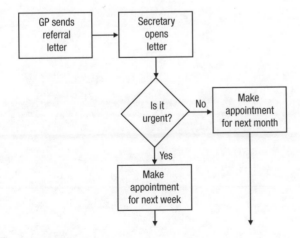

Hints and tips for using mapping decisions:

- Use the diamond shape as the tips will ensure you make the necessary links to activities in the process. (Square Post-it™ notes, rotated 45 degrees will give you a diamond shape.)
- If the decision takes you outside the boundaries of your process map, then put the activity in a circle (an ending). You can always come back to this and continue your map at a later date.
- Health care is very complex and there are always many decisions being made. Try to keep the decisions you map at a high level. This is usually sufficient to gain the benefits of mapping the process. Too many detailed decision points will make your map over complex.

Chapter 14
Make connections

Gillian was delayed in getting to the mapping meeting due to the upper GI clinic over running. It had not been a good day as they had difficulty in finding the clinical notes for three of the patients. In addition one of the patients wanted her daughter (her carer) to stay with her throughout the procedure, which slowed everything up.

When she arrived at the meeting her mood was no better. The team had split into two groups and had started finalising the map without her. One team had taken the decisions and activities and placed them in order on a piece of flipchart paper. They had put each Post-it™ note on the paper so they were touching each other. There was no space to draw connecting lines and the whole process didn't make sense, as the decision junctions weren't clear.

The other team, working on the beginning of the process, had done better. However, they were only part way through their diagram and because they had already drawn in all the lines and they had run out of paper, they had to start all over again.

Gillian took a deep breath and asked them to pause what they were doing so they could plan how to go about this stage of the mapping process.

This is the final stage of your mapping process. The purpose is to connect all the activities and decisions using arrows.

A bit of planning helps!

- Arrange the activities (rectangles) and the decisions (diamonds) on a piece of flipchart paper
- Join together flip chart paper or use newsprint rolls if your process map is a detailed one
- Only after you have arranged the pieces in an order you feel best reflects the process, should you draw in the lines
- Expect to discuss the order of the pieces and direction of the lines in the team
- Arrows can only be single headed and go in one direction (the patient can't move in two directions at the same time!)
- Don't worry about getting it perfect; there will always be ways to improve it
- Remember that what matters is what you learn about your process, not that you have a 'perfect' product in the form of a 'perfect' process map

Overcoming difficulties...

- Discussion and debate moves outside the boundaries, start and end point of the patient process the team agreed to map; *find your original process definition and refer the team to the details. If you find you do need to look outside the originally agreed definition, finish the current map first and then start a new one, agreeing the definition again etc.*
- Not completing the map: *you will probably never finish it to your liking so don't expect it to be finalised.*
- Focusing too much on the technical details of diagramming and losing sight of the purpose of mapping: *this is a delicate balance. It's useful to keep referring the team back to the reason for doing the map and to make notes on what you're learning. Make these notes explicit and encourage everyone to share their learning.*

Section C
Analysing

Mapping your process is the start of understanding what really happens to patients. Whilst it is possible to stop at mapping, if you carry out some further analysis you will discover new ways to make improvements and to reshape the patient's experience.

This section introduces a number of analytical tools and procedures that you can use separately, or you may find the greatest benefit is from spending a little time on each of them. They can generally be done in any order and your own project priorities should give you an indication which ones you would like to begin with.

There is no right or wrong way to analyse your process map. The benefit is in what you discover and then how you choose to resolve the issues and make the improvement.

**Ways of fixing problems often focus
only on 'treatment'**

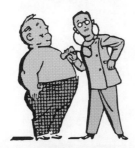

Always keep 'diagnosis' in mind

Each chapter will give you a **description of the topic** and some **explanation of how to go about the analytical process**. You may find alternative ways of conducting the analysis as this is only a guide and not a comprehensive 'how-to'. You may find you need more training or information about a particular issue, in which case you should approach the individuals and groups within your organisation who are geared up to provide this.

At the end of each chapter there are some **questions for redesign.** These are there to help you think about your analysis and to reflect how your process might be improved, taking the new information into account. Even if you don't carry out the analysis, you will find these questions useful for finding ways to reshape your process.

Chapter 15

Time

The general manager for the Medicine Department met with all the clinical nurse specialists to discuss the results of a survey of patient and carers recently completed by the hospital. This tied in with the organisation's annual objectives, many of which included improving waiting times for outpatient appointments and inpatient procedures. It was clear that the responses from patients were quite critical of the processes in the hospital and the requirement to improve was more than just meeting the national waiting list targets. Their complaints included the amount of time they waited to get an appointment, the time it took for a member of staff to answer the telephone when they had a query, the time they waited when they turned up for an appointment – in fact, to Gillian, it seemed like they complained of waiting for everything!

So time was a very important factor for the patient. Gillian thought about the process map they had just completed and wondered how they might use that to analyse the actual time each activity took as well as the elapsed time between activities and decisions. She did a quick mental calculation and she didn't like the answer. When the meeting finished she immediately called the mapping team together for a one-hour session with the aim of calculating the actual time spent on activities in the process, the elapsed time between activities as well as the total time it took for the whole process to be carried out – from the patient's perspective.

Agree on the common unit of time to use in your calculations: minutes, hours, days or weeks. This makes the calculations much easier to perform and to understand that there are different ways to think about time. Here are three:

Actual time

Each activity (rectangle) or decision (diamond) takes an amount of time to complete. *For example, "nurse preps patient – 8 minutes", "consultant carries out procedure – 22 minutes", "secretary types letter – 6 minutes".*

Elapsed time

This is the amount of time **between** each activity. *For example, "nurse preps patient",(5 minutes wait) "consultant carries out procedure",(102 minutes wait) "secretary types letter".*

Total time

Add actual time and elapsed time together and you will get the total time for the whole patient process. *For example, 8 + 5 + 22 + 102 + 6 = 143 minutes.*

% of time delivering care in the patient process

In the example given above, 36 minutes of activity took place over an elapsed time of 143 minutes. This means the 25% of the time in this process was actively engaging the patient – the rest may be considered wasted, especially from the point of view of the patient.

Questions to consider for redesign:

- What way can you reduce the unproductive waiting time between activities?
- Which decisions seem to slow the process down?
- Which activities took longer than you expected?
- Where is there variation in the amount of time taken per activity?
- What might help reduce this variation in time taken?

Chapter 16

Staff

Whilst the mapping team was putting the activities in sequence, Gillian spotted that there were far more people involved in the patient process than she had ever realised. In fact, when she last looked at the map she calculated there were twenty-eight different people involved from the time the GP made the decision to refer, to the time the report was returned to the practice. Some members of staff saw the same patient on at least three different occasions, on the same day! There was a lot of duplication. This fairly routine and straightforward patient process was proving to be one that kept many people very busy.

One of the advantages of the process map is its ability to make explicit what actually happens. Few people would guess that so many people are involved in one fairly simple patient process. The process map not only makes this evident but also helps you see where there is duplication of effort. Each of the following techniques will provide you with information from your map that you can use in any way that supports what you are trying to improve – the aim of your improvement project of which this mapping exercise is a part.

Who is involved in the process?

- Count the number of **roles** involved *e.g. nurses, doctors, secretaries*
- Count the number of **people** *e.g. there may be more than one consultant or secretary, so name them*

Your map may not contain sufficient detail to calculate this perfectly. However, the mapping team can easily brainstorm a list, filling in the detail as necessary.

Identify the duplications and double-backs

Note down where the patient sees the same person more than once, particularly if it is on the same day. Look for occasions where the process appears to go backwards because approval or more information is required from another person.

Top-down format

After you have drafted your map a useful technique is to draw up another map using the top-down format describe in chapter 9 using the key roles as headings. This will enable you, your mapping team and your work colleagues to get an overview of the complexity of the process. It also provides everyone with a sense of their role – where they fit into the process. This is useful to generate the tension for change.

Questions to consider for redesign:

- Which roles are central to the process? Why?
- Which people appear to have a greater contribution to the patient process than you anticipated? What are the implications of this?
- How can you remove the duplications and simplify the process?
- Who needs to be involved in the process that isn't – and who can be involved less than they are now? What are the implications for this?
- What activities could be carried out by different roles? Do these roles exist now?
- How many times is the patient handed from one health care professional to another?

Chapter 17

Place

When she started the process mapping exercise, Gillian never considered place to be something of importance or even worth analysing. She worked in the endoscopy suite and that is where the upper GI process took place – or so she thought. However, the process map had thrown up a whole series of issues, one of which was "place".

When they looked at what the patients actually experienced, it was clear their journey took them to a number of places that were geographically separate. For example, for some elderly patients with no transport, getting first to the GP surgery and then to the hospital was a complex process, often including the use of the ambulance trust's patient transport service. Even when they drove themselves to the hospital, the process map showed the parking allocated to the endoscopy patients was in fact further away than the endoscopy staff car park.

At a more detailed level, the endoscopy suite probably wasn't designed for good patient flow and efficiency. Confidential admission discussions were held on the open ward, the treatment rooms were at either ends of the ward which meant doctors and nurses wasted time moving between them.

"Place" – the space occupied by a person or a thing...

Health care services are constantly changing and developing. Most of the time, this means rearranging current space in the ward, adding new wings onto facilities, or shutting down other areas. There are seldom opportunities to design new services from a blank piece of paper. As a result there will be compromises made and some of these may, over time, end up impacting the patient's experience far more than was originally anticipated. In addition, some service may, by definition, be moved to and carried out in very different places. For example, some clinical procedures may end up being carried out in a primary care setting rather than the hospital.

Counting

You can count up the number of places at either a high level e.g. patient's home, GP surgery, hospital waiting room etc. or you can work at a more detailed level for parts of the process e.g. the various places around the endoscopy suit. At this detailed level you might find it useful to draw a plan of the work area and then draw lines showing how the patient and staff (use different colours for each) move around the space in carrying out the process.

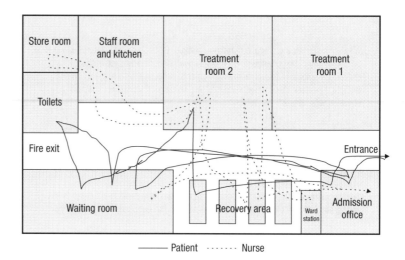

———— Patient   ······ Nurse

Top-down format

After you have drafted your map another useful technique, especially if you are working at the higher level, is to draw up another map using the top-down format described in chapter 9 using the *main places* where the process activities occur as the headings. This will enable you, your mapping team and your work colleagues to get an overview of the 'geography' of the process; namely the places to which the patient (or their proxy, such as information) travels. It also provides everyone with a sense of the whole of the process, especially the patient's view. This is useful to generate the tension for change (see opposite).

Questions to consider for redesign:

- Which activities appear not to be carried out in the place most appropriate for the patient?
- How does the design of the main work area affect the smooth flow of the process? What would you like to change and why?
- Can any of the activities be carried out in a different place altogether e.g. could the endoscopy be done at a community hospital close to the patient's home?

- How can space be freed up? What activities, if they were to stop, would create space that could be used for other tasks?
- How can you bring the places closer together so there is less time lost due to the patients or their information getting delayed in transit?
- How can new technology help improve the process? E.g. what will happen if information is transferred electronically?
- Which clinical activities are constrained to a specific place? Are there any trends to suggest that over time new clinical practices will have an impact on the space?

	GP consulting room in the practice	GP Secretary in the practice	Clinic Secretary in the departmental administrative wing	Patient's home
GP decides to refer				
GP Secretary prepares and sends letter to clinic				
Consultant's secretary receives letter via post room				
Consultant's secretary organises appointment				
Consultant's secretary sends patient letter giving date				
Consultant's secretary sends GP copy of letter				
Letter arrives with GP secretary				
GP receives information about the appointment				

Chapter 18

Resources

Gillian was getting into the swing of analysing her process map. She had completed the basics like finding out who was involved with what, when and where. Now she needed to have a look at the other resources being used by the process. Adrian had tipped her off that 'resources' as a topic for analysis was a useful one for finding ideas how to reduce the costs of the process, in terms of both the cash cost as well as other indirect costs – especially those incurred by the patient.

The general manager had recently asked for the departmental budget to be agreed for the next financial year. Gillian wondered whether the process map would provide a source of ideas for ways she could balance her budget for the endoscopy suite.

Adrian explained the most common understanding of 'resources' was staff costs and that was the basis for most budgets. However, he found that by focusing on the patient's process he found ideas to improve the management of things such as equipment and supplies. Gillian's non-staff items represented around 35% of her overall budget so she thought this would be a useful focus for some analysis.

You can use your process map to:

✓ Identify how you currently use equipment and supplies to support the activities
✓ Investigate which indirect resources you could access to help improve the process
✓ Discover how best to build on the patient's resources
✓ Find ways to manage the use of equipment and delivery of supplies that enables the flow of the patients through the process

Non-staff resources

- Equipment
- Supplies
- Indirect support e.g. audit, R&D, human resources, training

Patient's resources

- Primary carer
- Family and friends
- Religious organisations
- Voluntary organisations
- Information from books, the internet, from peers and family

Questions to consider for redesign:

- What plans can you make to ensure there are no delays created in the process due to a lack of available equipment or supplies?
- How can you best utilise indirect resources to help you reach your objectives?
- When considering the resources available to most of your patients, how could these be used to support their experience of the health care process you've mapped out?
- Which activities are dependent on the availability of equipment and supplies? What plan do you have to ensure that availability?

Chapter 19

Patient and carer views

So far Gillian had mapped the process from the patient's viewpoint but she had not performed any further analysis other than asking a couple of patients to check that the process map looked similar to the journeys they experienced. They both said that it did. One of the patients has shared the draft map with their son. He then wrote a long letter to Gillian explaining the difficulty he experienced with the process. For example, he had to park a long way from the endoscopy suite that meant looking for a wheelchair for his mother who couldn't walk very far and he had to take the whole afternoon off work, as the hospital couldn't give him a specific appointment time. He also complained about the fact that the hospital appointment arrived at short notice, disrupting his work schedule and that there was no information to explain to him or his mother about the procedure. As a result he had spent time searching the Internet for information and had found conflicting advice that was even less help. When he got his mother home she was unwell and he wasn't sure whom he was supposed to contact for advice – his GP or the hospital?

Gillian contemplated the list of ideas for improvement that the carer had supplied her with, and realised she needed to do some work to understand the patient's and carer's views of their experience.

Ask patients and carers:

❑ Which parts of the process do they feel work best? What do they want more of?
❑ If they could change three things about the process what would they be? Why?
❑ What ideas do they have to make the process smoother and more satisfactory?
❑ What do they think are the very small things that if changed will contribute to making a big difference to the experience?

Ways to involve patients and carers:

• Critical incident reviews (a formal process of interviewing someone to understand their experience and their perceptions of what occurred)
• Ask them questions, chat informally about the process, when they are in the waiting room

- Hold a focus group (discussion group of 6–9 individuals, usually led by facilitator, aimed at eliciting views and opinions on the process)
- Questionnaires – these can be very simple through to complex evaluations
- Follow up complaints
- Diaries; the patient records what happened to them and how they felt about it
- Tap into the patient representative groups and councils that exist at most hospitals and primary care practices

Please note: if you are involving patients or using their information, you need to check that you meet any ethics or research regulations laid down by your organisation.

Questions to consider for redesign:

- What are the most common complaints from patients? How can these be resolved by changing the process they experience?
- How can the patients' views be used to help build the tension and case for change amongst your colleagues – particularly those who may initially be unwilling to find new ways of working.

Chapter 20
Sequencing

Adrian's improvement team had made measurable improvements to their process for patients diagnosed with diabetes. Adrian explained to Gillian that one of the breakthroughs they had was when they started to think laterally about the different ways in which they could order the activities in the process.

Gillian made this topic a high priority for the next project meeting.

"Reordering activities can deliver improvements in the process"

The process that you have mapped out in *detail* provides you with a visual representation of what happens and in which order. What you do now is a reflection of the way in which the process has developed over time. No-one probably took the time to design it from scratch – it just sort of happened.

Now that you have completed your map you can focus on the sequence of events, the order in which things happen, and see whether there are any opportunities to reorder the activities, thus improving the overall patient experience.

An easy way to experiment with reordering the sequencing is to copy the activities onto Post-it™ notes, lay them out in the order of the current process, and then move them around. This way you will see the impact of any changes on the whole of the process. Different members of the mapping team can take copies of the activities and test out each of the questions below. Then, by combining and discussing your results, you may come up with some new and radical ideas on how to improve your process.

Questions to consider for redesign:

❑ What activities can you **eliminate** – stop doing altogether?
❑ What activities would benefit from **preparation ahead** of the time it is currently done? Especially if this means less effort and time taken at a later stage.
❑ Which ones can you **bring forward** to earlier in the process, especially if it means you reduce delays at a later stage?
❑ Which tasks can be done **in parallel** to others? How many different parts of the process can be done in parallel to reduce delays and dependencies?

❑ Which activities can be **automated** so that they happen more quickly and with less duplication or error?

❑ Can any of the tasks be **moved to a completely different stage** of the process?

❑ Which activities can be **done at a later** stage? Does this change in sequence really improve the patient's experience?

Chapter 21

Pareto analysis

The agenda at the mapping team meetings was becoming overwhelmed. There were many new ideas of what might be done to improve the process that the team was in danger of doing none of them, partly due to the difficulty in working out which one they should work with first. Apart from the prioritisation issue, how would they know which parts of the process, if redesigned, would have the most beneficial impact on the most patients?

Gillian realised they needed to do a similar analysis to the one they did in selecting their process (chapter 6) to find out where they would get the most improvement for their effort. They could use the similar "runners", "repeaters" and "specials" for parts for their process, that they had used to select it in the first place.

Adrian explained this was similar to pareto analysis and they would benefit from doing this exercise to check they were really working on the area with the largest opportunity for improvement, for the largest number of patients.

"80% of the problem is in 20% of the process"

Pareto analysis is a technique to discover where the largest problems, and therefore opportunities, lie in a process. It usually reveals that a small part of the process is responsible for most of the identified issues.

For example:

- 80% of delays are generated in 20% of the process
- 80% of incomplete referrals come from 20% of the general practitioners
- 20% of the process accounts for 80% of the value perceived by patients

Data are displayed as a bar chart that helps everyone see the main contributor to the problem (see opposite). This often means extra data collection, though you need only do this for those areas where you perceive a problem and where you would like to check where to target your efforts.

Incomplete referrals in last month (%)

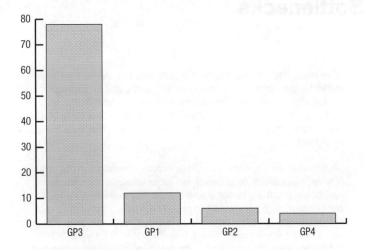

Questions to consider for redesign:

- Which aspect of the process contributes the most problems?
- Which areas should you avoid changing, as the overall impact for the patients and carers will be small?
- What additional data do you need to collect to demonstrate where you need to change?

Chapter 22

Bottlenecks

> Gillian noticed that whatever analysis they performed, they seemed to come up against the same problem every time when they were looking at how to speed up the flow of the patient through the process. It seemed they were short of a treatment room for about half of the week. There was no way they would be able to justify additional capacity so they would have to find ways of working around the problem.
>
> She discussed this with Adrian who said he discovered something similar in the diabetes project, though his bottleneck was not a treatment room, it was the availability of podiatrists. No matter what changes they planned and scenarios they calculated, they couldn't find a way to get rid of the problem. Instead, once they realised they had this constraint in the system, they changed the way they worked and the way the patient flowed, to ensure that when the podiatrist were in, they were utilised to the maximum. This meant finding ways to reduce patient "no-shows" and last minute cancellations.

"The process can only cope with the number of patients and at a speed that it's prime bottleneck can cope with – no more"

A bottleneck is a place in the process where the patients get delayed because the activity that is waiting to happen has some constraints that cannot be resolved. There is usually only one major bottleneck in a process. Many tasks look like they may be constraints but they are not. They may not be performing at their maximum capacity and this may be for a variety of reasons that can be solved e.g. using secure email to send back test results to the GP may solve what looked like a constraint – the secretary not having enough time to address, envelope and organise posting.

A good way to spot a bottleneck is when you see a large amount of work or patients queuing up waiting for something to happen. Think of the analogy of a dam holding back the water. If the water level gets very high, the floodgates can be opened. However, they are bottlenecks – only so much water can pass through them, no matter what you do. Therefore, if the dam keeps overflowing, the authorities need to find ways to divert the water. It is also in their interest, if the overflow is irregular, to keep a certain amount of water in the dam so that there is always some flowing through the floodgates. It is no good diverting the water so that another dam somewhere else experiences the same problem!

Living with the bottleneck

- Recognise the bottleneck for what it is and resolve to manage it well
- Make sure it is always operating efficiently and has minimum 'dead' time
- If it is equipment or facilities related, ensure maintenance is done out of hours or when patients are not demanding its use
- Reorganise and sequence the patient processes (and other related processes) to ensure the bottleneck is allowed to operate to maximise efficiency
- Continue to search for new and radically different ways to deliver the same process so the bottleneck can be relieved

Questions to consider for redesign:

- Where is the one critical activity in the process where the capacity defines the amount and rate of patient throughput?
- How can you ensure the bottleneck operates to maximum efficiency?

Chapter 23

Value

The debate at the mapping and departmental team meetings was becoming more intense. It appeared that everyone was committed to making improvements in the patient's process, however, each person thought their bit of the process was the most important and, of course, there was little wrong with it. Gillian was struggling to find a way that kept the focus on the patient's experience in practice, as well as theory.

Adrian suggested she might like to find a way that differentiated between the activities the patient valued and the ones they didn't care about. This would keep the discussion focused on the patient's view and at the same time highlight those activities and delays that were not valued by the patient.

What about those activities the patient didn't feel contributed directly to their care but were a necessary part of maintaining a service; for example, training and record keeping? Adrian reassured Gillian that this exercise wasn't about judging whether something is right or wrong, or whether it should be done or not. It is really about thinking through and discovering ideas where making changes in everyday practice may deliver a real and measurable improvement that patients and staff can recognise.

"Value – what the patient perceives to be worthwhile"

"Value" is a subjective and emotional term. Of course, all the tasks that are carried out by someone are deemed to be useful, else why would they be doing them? One of the benefits of process mapping is that it enables all those involved to see a wider view of their involvement and contribution to patient care. Because clinical and administrative support requirements are changing all the time, processes and procedures tend to just happen along the way, without design. The advantage of stepping back and thinking about how the patient values different activities in the process, allows you to see where you can make radical changes to improve how you deliver their care.

Ways to think of the value of activities from the patient's perspective:

1. **Adds value**; the patient perceives that this is the core reason for their contact with health care services. For example, undergo a test or have a consultation with the consultant
2. **Limited value**; the patient sees the activities as not directly contributing their care. For example, the activities involved

in booking an appointment or having to repeat their personal history every time they encounter a health professional

3. **Limited value but necessary**; the best judge of this is the health practitioner or manager. This covers things like training and data collection for audit purposes

Analysing value in your mapped process:

The temptation is to agree most of your activities add value, a large number have limited value but are operationally necessary, and very few are of limited value. Your challenge is constructively, to be critical and thought provoking. Try for no more than 25% of your current process to be identified as adding value and less than 30% as limited value but necessary.

An easy way to facilitate the discussion is to go about it in two rounds, firstly to separate "*adds value*" from "*limited value*", and then to take the limited value activities and see which are still necessary operationally.

Copy the main activities from your process map onto Post-it™ notes. Then arrange these on a flip chart as in the example below. Start by placing the notes on the centre line and then discuss each one, deciding where to place it on the chart.

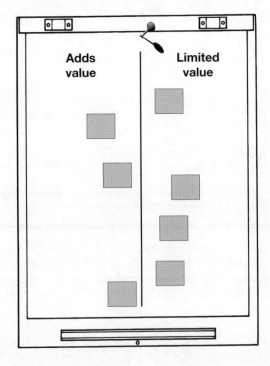

This process needs careful facilitation. The participants need to be reassured that no one is judging their performance or saying their job needs to go. Yes, there are many implications in what is discussed; however, it is important to remind everyone that this is primarily an analytical exercise to help them learn about their process. Keeping the patient's focus to the fore should help. You may also find it useful to test your findings with a group of patients and carers.

Questions to consider for redesign:

- What activities are low on the 'value' list for both patients and staff?
- Which activities do patients value? How do you know?
- How can you improve a 'limited value' activity (as perceived by the patient) that you need to retain for operational purposes? Are you sure you need to keep the activity in its current form?
- Which of the 'limited value but necessary' activities can be improved so they add value? For how long will they remain necessary?

Chapter 24

Waste

The mapping process and the analyses they had started to do, demonstrated to the mapping team that many of the activities that were carried out in fact were quite wasteful. One of the team members, Zola, wanted to see if taking the focus of 'waste' in their process would highlight any new areas for improvement.

Gillian was concerned that some people would see this as a cost cutting exercise. Zola explained that of course there was a financial implication but this was not the purpose of the exercise. She explained that as a manager in the sterile services department, she was aware of many different things that were happening in the upper GI process that she thought were wasteful. Even the way equipment was moved around could be wasteful. In doing this process map she could see that her services were not necessarily designed to support Gillian's endoscopy services.

It was agreed they would spend a couple of hours analysing waste in their process, and Zola volunteered to lead what she hoped would be a light-hearted and informative process. In the end it turned out alright, though Zola had to work hard to make sure that no-one got defensive about waste that just happened to involve them or be in their area of work.

"Waste – the patient's perspective is crucial"

One way to discover waste is to take each of the following types of waste and to list where you think this happens in your process. It is useful to describe why you think it happens and to start to gather ideas on how to remove or reduce it. You will find some of these types of waste overlap, giving you sometimes four or five reasons (all of them about waste) to improve your process.

You can work through the list as a whole team, or you can divide up the types of waste amongst the team members for analysis and then ask them to report back to the whole group.

It is possible, and desirable, to spend no more than an hour discovering the key areas and types of waste in your process. Once you have identified where the biggest problems are (the 80/20 of the Pareto process described earlier), then you can work on those parts of the process in more detail.

Types of waste

1. **Waiting**; this occurs whenever time is not being used effectively. Time is important for patients, carers, staff and equipment. Whilst you can put a cost on this, the best unit for analysis is time itself – use minutes, hours or days. Investigate the time wasted and check the knock on impact for all people involved in the process.

2. **Transporting**; chasing appointments at different places can be wasteful for both patients and staff. Look for unnecessary journeys and movements between locations. Count the locations and check whether there are alternative ways to deliver the service. How many times does the patient attend the hospital or surgery and can a number of activities be combined into the same visit?

3. **Unnecessary motion**; at a more detailed level, the design of the workplace can create wasteful movements. Seek opportunities to place tasks closer together. Check how often one person repeats a movement or appears to keep going back to where they have just come from. How can you alter the physical environment or the policies and procedures so this can be reduced?

4. **Over processing**; this happens when you do more activities than necessary; for example, carrying out too many tests. Over complicating processes and tasks is wasteful. What needs to happen to reduce the inappropriate overuse of some resources? What ideas does this give you for redesigning your patient process?

5. **Unnecessary inventory**; where systems are unreliable, extra stock is often ordered and held 'just in case'. This is wasteful not only in terms of cost, but also storage space. Discover why you have such large stocks. Which systems and processes that impact your patient process need to be investigated to ensure your activities run as smoothly as possible? How will you go about resolving these issues?

6. **Re-work**; repeating a task because it wasn't completed properly the first time is very wasteful. Do you know where the most errors seem to happen? How can you find out? What are the reasons for these happening? What can you do to resolve these?

What changes to the process would help reduce the amount of re-work that happens in the process?

7. **Untapped human potential**; this means not making the most of the skills and abilities of members of staff as well as patients and their carers. How can you find out who has skills not being used? Which job roles can be extended to enable greater use of an individual's abilities? Who might benefit from a little training to bring out the best in them? What are your plans to develop the competences and capabilities of all those involved in the process – including patients and carers?

8. **Under-utilised resources**; expensive equipment and facilities that are used for only a few hours a day are wasteful. The usual focus is that there isn't enough resources to do what you need to do. However, this type of waste forces you to consider which nonhuman resources you don't work efficiently. For example, for how many hours is the new MRI scanner used over the 168 hours in the week? What might you do to ensure resources are available for the patient process for as long as possible? What needs to change for this to happen?

What do you need to do with waste? – get rid of it! Or at the very least, reduce it. Yes, it's an emotional concept and one person's waste may be another person's treasured task. The benefit of this activity is in looking at waste from the *patient's perspective*. Keep that focus at all times and you'll find new ideas on how to transform your process.

Chapter 25

Demand

Adrian mentioned to Gillian that he was now working on how they could better manage the demand for diabetes services. Gillian was intrigued as she felt that was an issue not in the control of the hospital. Adrian took her through some of the principles and ways he was assessing demand for his service. He also explained that to do the job properly you had to do a lot more extra work, some of which may be more than the original mapping team was set up to do. He recommended she do a little analysis, and then if they felt they could influence the demand, then to call together another team who could work specifically on demand and capacity.

Gillian could see Adrian's point, however, she felt she could do a lot more with her mapping team and was determined to have a go. It was obvious that just working out how many patients they saw on average, each day, would be useful. Some of the mapping team thought this was a waste of time and their job was to meet any demand that came their way – how could you work out the average for emergencies? Gillian explained that even emergencies weren't infinite and that by finding the range of numbers of patients who underwent an endoscopy, urgent or routine, then they could make better plans.

"Demand is not infinite"

Demand is an input into your process. It is the reason why you do it – because others have requirements of you. For convenience, demand is often categorised into urgent, soon or routine. However, putting demand in a category doesn't make it go down or be dealt with any quicker – it may even slow up the whole process due to the inefficient use of resources. A lot of demand issues may appear to be outside your control. However, an efficient process where the patient experiences a reliable service (i.e. no hospital-initiated cancellations) is one that smooths out the numbers being seen in any clinic; it operates to a regular beat and copes with surprises.

The primary demand in any process is the number of patients to be seen. One of the first tasks in understanding demand is to discover what your current demand is like. This may be different from the actual numbers of patients seen; for example, some referrals (primary demand) may be referred on and dealt with elsewhere. In this case you would not be satisfying your true demand, so try to capture data that will find these anomalies for you.

Calculating the demand for your process

- How many patients go through your process in a week, a month, a year?
- Where does this demand come from? GP referrals, walk in clinics, other wards in the hospital?
- What are the patterns in demand?
- What are the most common ranges for demand e.g. GP referrals appear to be between 15 and 20 every week, with a dip in the summer months.

Questions to consider for redesign:

- What action can you take to smooth demand? How can you get rid of the regular peaks and troughs in the numbers of patients that go through your process?
- Check of 'perverse' incentives that may increase demand e.g. policies
- Identify and remove barriers to smoothing demand

Chapter 26

Capacity

Right from the start of the process mapping exercise, the team had been swamped with demand from their colleagues for more nurses, more technicians, more equipment and more space. Even some of the team believed the only way to improve the patient's experience was to make more capacity available for the upper GI process.

Adrian had already warned Gillian that this would happen. He also explained that when they added an extra diabetes nurse it actually made their patient process worse. The reasons was she added a lot more complexity to the system and it meant they didn't look at areas they could improve – they just made the assumption she would make the process better. In the end, they reshaped their process and she ended up taking a new course and moving into another area in the hospital.

Gillian thought a good place to start assessing whether they had a genuine need to increase capacity was to calculate what they already had. She wanted to know the potential they had for the upper GI process. The next step would then be to check whether the process was using the capacity in the most efficient way, or whether the process itself was wasting resources.

"Adding more capacity than the process needs may worsen the patient's experience"

Capacity is the amount of resources available for a process. Usually resources are shared by a number of separate processes and it is useful to calculate the total of the resources available, then work out how much is currently used by the process and how much spare or shortfall there is.

Work out what capacity you have in total

- Staff; list the various roles and note the total number of hours they are available for work in a week, excluding time for training, audit etc.
- Equipment/procedure room; list the rooms or items of equipment and work out the total number of hours that they are available in a week (regardless of staffing issues). You should note when equipment/rooms are idle so use the 24 hour clock. Remember to deduct time for maintenance and cleaning.

What is the available capacity for your process?

Using the total capacity you identified above, calculate how much is available for your process. Keep equipment/rooms separate from staffing as this will help you identify where the constraints may lie. Take into account the number of people required per procedure and work out how long the average procedure takes to complete.

Identify what capacities the patient may have e.g. can they perform some of the preparation safely at home? Also list the capacity elsewhere that could be supportive to the process e.g. Community hospitals

Questions to consider for redesign: matching capacity to demand

- Check the demand for the process (chapter 25) and see how it matches up to your potential capacity.
- Discuss the mismatches and come up with ideas on how to resolve them by redesigning your process, before you add capacity
- If you do need to add capacity, can this be done by freeing up or redeploying existing resources, before you bring new staff or equipment into the process?

Section D

Taking action

After you have mapped and analysed your process you will have many ideas on how to improve your process. Now you need to get down to some action – implementing the proposed changes.

There is no right or wrong way to implement changes to a process. You will have a good understanding of your own local context, and that is what matters. Implementation strategies that work for one team may not work for yours. So, instead of offering you a formula for implementing change, this section provides you with some guidance in key areas.

The next chapter on **redesigning** gives you some hints and tips on getting started in the redesign process. It is important you do some planning, and this includes mapping what the new process could look like.

"Pulling" and "pushing" are terms used to describe the manner in which patients are moved through the process. This chapter is designed to get you thinking about how you can find ways to reduce the amount of pushing and replace it with the patient being called and attracted into the next stage of the process. Push type processes often have long delays and more unnecessary administration than 'pull' type processes.

In **roles and skills** there are ideas on how you can use the untapped potential amongst staff members as well as patients and carers. This includes developing new roles as well as identifying training opportunities.

How will you know whether the process you have redesigned is better than the average performance for similar processes? The chapter on **benchmarking** suggests you spend a little time assessing how your processes compares to those carried out in other organisations.

Patient feedback will have been an integral part of your mapping process. In this chapter you are guided to consider how you can maintain patient and carer involvement in the continuous development and improvement of your process.

The changes you make will have some form of impact on **clinical outcomes**. Working through what these might be, whether they are what you anticipate or not, and ways to manage any difficulties is covered in this chapter.

Finally, there are some thoughts on how you **maintain flexibility** in the solution you are implementing. Rigid procedures are difficult to sustain in an environment that is constantly changing. The last chapter in this section encourages you to consider the changes that will happen anyway and to carry out some scenario planning to let you see how you might best respond.

Chapter 27

Redesigning

By now the upper GI team had completed their process map and performed a number of analyses, all of which provided them with a long list of potential ideas on how to improve the patient's experience of the process. They were ready to start redesigning their process.

Gillian had been holding them back from making changes until they had completed most of the analytical work. The reason for this was to make sure they didn't start making changes in one place that had a negative knock on impact in another. Whilst it would never be possible to work it all out she felt a good place to start could be by drawing a process map of the new process. Gillian felt it was important the team all had a common understanding of what the new process would look like and that they could use this to guide the implementation of the changes.

The mapping team spent much longer on the design phase of their new process than they anticipated. Some of the participants really wanted to change things quickly, but once they understood the complexities of thinking through and designing a new process they realised the importance of planning. This was especially as the process they were working on was only one of many in their department. It was clear that their changes would have an impact on other processes and they needed to take these into account in their own work.

"At last – you can map the new process!"

Summarising your current process

- List the issues, constraints, problems with the process
- List your ideas on how to resolve the issues
- Match up the issues with the ideas and check for completeness; don't worry whether the ideas are practical or not at this stage. You may have many ideas to resolve one type of issue

Mapping the new process

- Draw a high level map of the proposed new process
- Assess how it differs from the current process and note the implication of this
- Identify the areas of most change
- Map these areas in more detail
- Again, assess the differences from the current process and the implications of this

Project planning

- Choose which changes you intend to make in the short term, and set aside those that require influence beyond your control at this time
- Decide which changes have the longest lead time and make plans on how to begin the work on these
- List at least 15 very small changes that you can start making NOW.

The change process is best carried out through very small cycles of change, doing one tweak, seeing whether it had the desired effect, then doing another. This way you can test whether your ideas were good ones and also encourage others to change by encouraging them to take small steps rather than feel overwhelmed by a significant step change. (See annotated bibliography – "The Improvement Guide" for more information on this way to deliver improvements.)

Chapter 28

Pulling and pushing

When they reviewed their process with a group of patients and carers, the mapping team was challenged to think about the ways in which the interaction between patients and staff influenced the experience of everyone involved. One of the patients, a production manager at the local furniture factory, mentioned that he felt he was pushed from one part of the health service, one department, one nurse, to another. He said he bore the brunt of that pushing around as the new person or place he went to greet him with a sigh as if he was adding to the complexity of their day. The one time this didn't happen was when the nurse called him from the waiting room to the procedure room. He said it felt like he was being pulled along the process that was more comfortable for him. He explained this was not unlike the processes they employed in his factory. There they tried to find ways where someone down the line pulled the jobs towards them, rather than being recipients of what felt like others' work being dumped on them. He said this not only made the process feel better for all involved, but was also more efficient.

Gillian remembered this and thought it might be useful for the team to assess their new process and see how much pulling versus pushing was going on. She asked the patient if he wouldn't mind facilitating this session for them. He was delighted to help.

Key questions for your newly designed process are:

- **Why does the push strategy exist in the first place?** Look at your process and discuss why it is that patients are pushed to and through the various activities. What is the reason for this? Who is the reason? What are the implications for changing this?

- **To what extent can you pull the patient through the process?** What ideas do you have to call the patient into the next activity? Who needs to help make this happen?

- **Which activities can proactively ask for the next patient (or piece of equipment)?** This is not dissimilar to carrying out preventative maintenance on a piece of equipment. You can either wait for it to go wrong and then demand a repairman, or you can keep the equipment operating at peak performance by regular maintenance.

- **How can you synchronise steps in the process?** This means you need to find a way to manage the variation between activities and tasks. Are you considering the demand and capacity at each stage in the process? What automated or semi-automated methods can you put in place to make sure the patient's path is smooth and swift, with the connections between steps hardly noticed?

- **At which point in your process does the pull turn to push?** Whilst the aim is to have as much pull in the process as possible, sometimes push is unavoidable. How far up the process can you move the pull? Investigate the points at which push and pull change; what's going on here and how can you improve the interface?

Chapter 29

Roles and skills

Gillian realised that the majority of the changes to the process would mean staff changing the ways they work. For some people this was a small procedural modification of the way they carried out their duties. However, for others there were significant implications. Even to the extent that some roles could change so much that they would need to be re-evaluated by the human resources department, regraded and new job descriptions agreed.

Similar experiences happened in the diabetes department when they redesigned their processes. In fact they ended up with a new role that combined a number of tasks previously carried out by separate members of staff. For example, taking blood samples (used to be the phlebotomist' role), measuring blood pressure (used to be the clinical nurse specialist) and checking the patient's blood glucose diary (not done by anyone) were now done by a new nursing assistant role. Adrian explained this was preferred by the patient and freed up other nursing staff to spend more time with patients discussing their issues in more detail.

"Do what you've always done
– and you'll get what you've always got."

The big leap

If you could create new roles for your newly designed process, what would they be? How can the process be reshaped and improved by changing who carried out which task? If you were starting from a blank sheet of paper, how would you design the health care roles? These questions are designed to make you think about the opportunity for restructuring roles. You will encounter many reasons why these changes can't be implemented, however, creating a vision of what might be possible is an important step in the redesign process. To deliver a real improvement you will need to find new ways of carrying out the process.

Developing new roles takes time and there are many hurdles along the way. Some professions may require certain minimum standards and procedures if anything is to be changed. These are in place to ensure good care for the patient, though you should not be afraid to challenge professional assumptions, to make sure they are keeping up with the times. If you believe you will be trying to change staff roles, then you need to involve your human resources department early on in the process.

Practicalities

- List the roles covered in your process map and identify what new ways of working they will need to implement in order for your newly designed process to work most effectively
- What new roles are you expecting patients and carers to adopt?
- Assess whether any other processes will be impacted by the proposed changes in duties, tasks and roles.
- Discuss these changes and their implications with the staff, patients and carers involved in the process.
- If you have brand new roles, then work closely with the human resources department and the relevant professional organisations. You may need to pilot and test how the new role will work.
- Identify what training is required. Plan for it.
- Most roles adapt over time and outgrow their job descriptions. Keep testing and stretching – keep involving people and finding ways to use their true capacity.

Chapter 30

Benchmarking

The general manager responsible for the endoscopy department challenged the mapping teams newly designed process. He wanted to know how they knew this was one of the best ways to do it. Gillian explained there was probably no right or wrong way of delivering a patient process and they had designed one that they felt solved most of the issues they identified at the start of the project. The general manager was not entirely convinced. He was concerned that other organisation were doing similar improvement projects and he had heard some of them were achieving significant measurable improvement – greater than what Gillian's team anticipated.

Gillian explained that she understood his position, however, their process map took into account the specific circumstances in the organisation. Their context was their own and she wasn't sure that what worked somewhere else would work for them.

The general manager agreed with Gillian and understood her point of view. However, he was adamant that they test out their new process with at least two other organisations, to ensure they had really come up with a solution that was top class, amongst the best possible.

Benchmarking is a way of learning from others and making sure your solutions are keeping up with what others are implementing or already delivering. You can also benchmark your current process to see just how far away you are from the processes delivered by leading organisations.

The process of benchmarking your process need not take a long time. Some benchmarking studies are complex and conducted over many years. In this case, you are looking to carry out a small pragmatic exercise as part of your improvement project. You may find your audit department can help you.

Why benchmark

❑ Identify improvement goals that stretch your idea of improvement
❑ Discover ways to deliver improvement
❑ Test whether your potential solutions are the best possible

Planning to benchmark

- Decide **what** it is you would like to benchmark; the current process or the newly designed one. Which parts of the process?
- **With whom** can you benchmark. It is useful to do this with organisations of similar size and population base. However, you might also choose to test yourself against leading organisations that are very different as you may discover ideas on how to improve your process that have nothing to do with the size or nature of the organisation. You should seek out places where they are recognised as delivering an excellent service.
- **When** should you do it? A good time is before you finalise your newly designed process and begin implementing changes.

Observing and learning

- One of the best ways to benchmark is to visit the other organisations. You can follow a patient through their process, checking what happens against your current or new process map.
- Compare your process to that of the other organisations. List the differences and test whether you need to update your newly designed process.

Chapter 31

Patient feedback

> Earlier when they started analysing their process, the mapping team learnt just how valuable were the patient and carer views on their process (see chapter 19). Already a number of changes had been made to the upper GI process and they wanted to put in place some system where they could continue to get feedback from patients and carers.
>
> They contacted Adrian to find out what he had put in place in the diabetes process. He explained that he had been remiss in this area, and wished he had done a lot more. He felt this project team made a lot of changes that they found out later were not sustainable or didn't actually solve the initial problem. Usually it was patients who pointed this out. He wished they had set up some way to validated and check their actions with patients and carers. Gillian asked for help from the person responsible for improving processes in the organisation. He suggested she design some simple questionnaires that could be assessed by the staff at the end of each clinic. He also thought that the occasional focus group would be helpful.

"Feedback must be received at the point of service delivery"

The patient's viewpoint is easily forgotten once the project has been completed and some improvements made. You started mapping your process from the patient's perspective and it is important you continue to reflect this in the ongoing assessment of the process. Different members of staff working in different stages of the process will probably want different types of feedback.

Designing feedback

- **What** topics or activities would make the best focus?

- **How often** should feedback occur? Of course there is feedback at every patient encounter – just watch the body language and listen to what is said. But you can also develop systems to capture feedback after every clinic (best), or every week. Once feedback is separated in time from the event, the opportunities for learning diminish.

- **Which method** would be appropriate and pragmatic? Short questionnaires that can be completed in the waiting room are helpful. You could give every fifth patient one or two questions about the process they have experienced so far, and record the responses in a log for others to read. There are many different methods. The key factor is to keep it simple and easy so that it gets done without too much effort and becomes part of every-day working practice.

- **Reviewing and reporting**; sometimes it is helpful to get the department together to review the patient's responses. This could be done on a regular basis and is very effective when it involves all members of the process, including those who may be from outside your immediate organisation. On the other hand, don't let formal reporting get in the way of individuals and teams gaining quick responses to the care they are delivering. That way they get confirmation they are doing the right thing or they can take immediate action to improve the process if that is necessary.

Chapter 32

Clinical outcomes

> Gillian was concerned that they had altered the criteria for the referral of patients for an upper GI endoscopy. No-one else seemed concerned but she was worried that they may be missing some patients that they used to get, and getting some patients that still should not be part of the upper GI process. She discussed this with some colleagues and they all said she should ask the audit department to do some sort of evaluation in 12 or 18 months time.
>
> Gillian was not happy to wait that long so she thought she would build in a review system for the project changes and then use the regular departmental meeting to discuss any anomalies or concerns.

The patient process is primarily about flow; the way in which a patient moves though the health care system. Whilst you will have taken clinical considerations into account when you designed your solution, it is worth taking a little time to check the impact the changes may have had on clinical outcomes.

To some extent this is a discipline in its own right! The objective here, as part of your mapping exercise and improvement project, is do carry out a pragmatic review to ensure there are no known negative implications of the changes you have made, or are about to make.

If you have gone about the change process using small cycles of change (chapter 27) then you will have already reduced the risk of any significant problem. However, you may have a creeping error; this is something that is very small when you find one of them, but over time it tends to expand and become more of an issue. For example, the way a referral is worded could include some patients that previously were not part of the process. Over time, this could increase demand on your process and could also mean that patients undergo unnecessary procedures.

Review the clinical impact of changes

- Will the changes mean different patients will be seen? What are the implications of this?
- Do we expect the clinical outcomes to be different after we have changed the process? Will they be better or worse? Why?

- Which members of the health care team feel there will be a negative impact on clinical outcomes? What are their concerns?
- How can you check the impact on clinical outcomes without waiting months for a full audit review?
- What needs to happen to implement your ideas for the above?
- What data will be useful to collect at the point of service delivery? How can this be turned into quick and regular feedback e.g. using automated systems and graphs?

Chapter 33
Maintaining flexibility

Adrian was having problems keeping some of his changes going. He thought he had put in place agreed procedures that were sufficiently detailed and tied into the day-to-day operation of the diabetes clinic. However, he was discovering that it was those things that he thought he had fixed and frozen into the system that appeared to give him the most problems.

Gillian suggested to him that perhaps it was because everything was so rigid and sorted that the process was becoming difficult to sustain. She explained to Adrian that the role descriptions and all the rules and regulations meant there was very little flexibility in his redesigned process. This meant that when small changes happened, such as a key member of staff being off ill, the whole process was at risk because there were no easily applied alternatives.

"Sustainability – the ability to continue to co-evolve
with the changing environment"

The end of your project is certainly not the end of the improvement work on your process. You will continually have demands on you to keep changing. Nothing ever stands still and certainly, there will be new professional regulations, new clinical technologies, new patient demands and other new demands from people, places and organisations you haven't yet thought about!

In the same way that a rigid structure may be broken by the wind, procedures may lack the flexibility to adapt to the pressures that will come their way. It is important that you not only implement supple solutions but that you also spend some time with your team working out what the pressures are likely to be and then carrying out some scenario planning – what if this happens, what if that happens…

What will continue to be the pressures for change?

- Brainstorm all the pressures and demands that will be on your process
- Prioritise these
- Assess the impact on the process (significant, major, minor, little)
- Assess the likelihood of them happening (% probability)

- Note the timescale when you expect some things might be impacted

Scenario planning

Using the information you have gathered from the section above, work out what are the three most likely scenarios and write brief descriptions of them. Use these as the basis for discussion with your team and other important participants in the process.

The objective is NOT to work out how to stop the pressures happening; most of them will happen anyway, and even more will happen that you don't know about! Instead, spend some time discussing how you will cope with some of the possible changes. Test whether your newly designed process has a built in capability to adjust automatically and with little fuss to the types of pressures that you expect to experience on a regular basis e.g. staff sickness.

Every time you ask "what if…" you are preparing yourself for some of the changes that will happen. The more you do this, the more you can test the adaptability of the process and prepare yourself, and others, for the fact that things will change – anyway.

Section E

Facilitating

As a facilitator, your role is twofold:

✓ To help others in your team carry out the task of mapping, analysing and improving the patient process
✓ Improving the way the team members work with each other and the rest of their colleagues involved in delivering the patient process.

You will need to be thinking about four different areas:

1. **Task**: *the work you and your team need to do to achieve the objectives of the mapping and improvement exercise.* One of your roles is to clarify and explain the tasks to team members. This includes showing how all the activities will fit together to achieve the project objectives.
2. **Process**: *what needs to happen, in what way, to achieve the task.* You will need to be an active listener and help your team members work together to plan what they should do, solve problems and complete their tasks.
3. **Team dynamics**: *what is happening amongst your team members, how the interactions between individuals are impacting on the project.* You will need to manage conflict that arises and use a variety of personal skills to build a cohesive and productive team.
4. **Self**: *how your behaviour influences the team.* You need to understand about your own learning and managing styles, and the impact these have on others. You can use your personal abilities to influence the team.

This section provides you with some guidance on how to organise your team and your mapping exercise, how to keep discussion flowing, ways of coping with those difficult moments that will occur and how you can acknowledge and value different points of view.

This is not a comprehensive guide to facilitation. You already have significant experience and skills in this area – anyone who is working in health care will already have developed some abilities to facilitate complex situations.

The best way to learn how to facilitate teams and improvement projects is to practice. Over time your own style will develop. Keep a learning diary and reflect on what is working well for you, and build on it. Identify any specific learning needs you may have and access suitable learning opportunities.

Chapter 34

Organising and supporting

> The upper GI improvement project had been finished for about six months. The results were still good and the team was continuing to make small changes. Gillian was asked to attend a workshop with other Clinical Nurse Specialists to share her experience of facilitating the mapping exercise.
>
> Most of the nurses seemed to be interested in how she managed to carry out the mapping whilst still doing her regular nursing job. Gillian explained she was released for two sessions per month and a locum CNS was provided so her clinical work could continue without too much difficulty. However, she made it clear that it was very important that she was well organised. The mapping exercise produces lots of papers, ideas, notes from meetings, meetings them-selves – all of which needed analysing and synthesising. She also tried to keep the meetings as short and productive as possible as many of the team members had clinical roles. This meant each meeting had to be well planned and prepared.
>
> Gillian explained that she had learnt how to delegate. It was not possible for her to do the mapping exercise. All the team members had to participate. She encouraged them to give some time and use the skills they had to contribute to the process. Some team members were able to use skills they did not use in their regular work. For example, one of the consultants turned out to be developing, in his spare time, computer programmes to support audit. He developed a few useful spreadsheets that were used in analysing the upper GI map.

If you are responsible for the mapping exercise then you will need to **design a system to help you manage all the tasks that you may be required to do**. The list below suggests where you can start:

- Read through Section A: Getting Started in this book and note what you need to do to produce a process map
- Work out how you will communicate with team members; if on email then develop a group list, if by letter then print some labels, if by telephone, then make sure you have access to a phone and agree times when best to contact each person (you might also like to have an answering machine)
- Find space in your office (or somebody else's office!) where you can store your papers and draft maps. These will often be on flipcharts so you might like to buy a cardboard roll to keep them in (flipcharts have the habit of "disintegrating" during storage!)
- Sort out a filing system in a couple of lever arch files where you can store all your notes and analyses. As mapping is not a lin-ear process, you will find lots of ideas being discussed at times

when you really don't want to deal with them. You need to be able to capture and store those ideas so you can go back to them later.

Supporting and delegating

- Ensure the members of your mapping team are clear about what is expected of them. Find out what they can contribute and discuss with each of them, the level of commitment you anticipate.
- For many on the team this will be an unfamiliar process working with people they usually don't meet. You may find it useful to contact each member quite frequently, especially after meetings, to see whether they need any support from you. It is preferable that you delegate the ownership of the task to someone else and then support them doing it, than try and do it all yourself.

Chapter 35
Holding the conversation

Throughout the mapping exercise, Gillian was surprised at the amount of debate that was generated. This was regardless of what stage they were at – it just seemed like everyone had a lot to say, all the time! She noticed that all team members were engaged in seeing the whole process and in discovering their part in it.

Creative ideas on how to resolve the problem were always coming up. When they were trying to maintain the focus on the current situation, Gillian made notes of the ideas, told everyone that she had heard and recorded the idea, and then stored it for use later on. This was helpful in maintaining a focus on the current process as the tendency was to rush and make changes as soon as they had any ideas. By slowing down the actions and spending a bit more time deliberating and discussing the changes they could make, Gillian felt they ended up with better and more sustainable solutions.

"Discussion around the map is more important than the map itself"

It is easy to believe that the output of the process mapping exercise is the map itself, and possibly also the various analyses you carry out. However, the most important and productive output from the process is the personal and team learning that it produces. It is the discussion around the mapping process that matters most. Individuals who participate in the mapping exercise will discover what actually happens, from the perspective of the patient, in the process under review. They will find out things they may have preferred not to know and have the opportunity to discuss these difficult issues.

Balance the discussion

The discussion around tricky issues is important and should be encouraged. At times this may be challenging and you may prefer to avoid this and focus on the production of the map. Whilst you will need to find a balance between mapping and discussing, and indeed, without the map there is little to discuss, you should pay careful attention to how you facilitate and enable conversation about what the map is showing.

Capturing creative thoughts

The really creative ideas for improving process tend to appear when analysing the process and arguing over what it all means. A flippant remark, something surprising, something that makes you laugh – these are all hints that what has been said might be very creative. If this happens, then pause, draw attention to the idea and then explore it a bit further. It may have been an unrealistic thought, however, with some probing, tweaking and development, it may turn into an exciting new way of working.

Active listening

One of the best ways to support and enable conversation

- ✓ **Encouraging** – to show interest and keep the person talking: use non-committal words such as *"I see...", "That's interesting..."*
- ✓ **Restating & reflecting** – to show you're listening and demonstrate you have grasped the issue: restate the basic ideas, *"If I understand your idea is...", "In other words...", "You feel that..."*
- ✓ **Summarising** – to pull together ideas and facts, review progress: *"These seem to be the key ideas expressed...", "If I understand, you feel this way about ..."*

Chapter 36
Difficult moments

At the workshop for colleagues who were about to start similar mapping exercises, Gillian was asked when she experienced the most difficulties; at what points in the process did she have the most problems.

Gillian was cautious in answering this and explained that she felt each project would be quite different as the skills of the project leader, facilitator and team members would all be different. Also the context in which they were working would be different for each team and organisation. However, there were a few incidents that she thought others might experience so she shared these.

When asked her advice on how to resolve these again, Gillian said she felt that it would be down to whom each leader would like to deal with in the local circumstances. She was reluctant to give too much advice on how to resolve problems, but explained to them how she went about it.

The 'difficult moments' listed below are those that most mapping teams will experience. Your team may not experience any of these, but if you do, you need to know that it is expected. Or you may experience different issues, again, this list is not comprehensive so you should expect some to happen that are not covered here.

❑ At the start; gaining commitment to join the mapping team, describing why it is a worthwhile exercise
❑ How and when to involve patients and carers in the exercise
❑ First team meeting; introducing each other, what do we call each other, why are you here, why am I here…
❑ Defining the process; agreeing the start and end points of the process, and what is excluded
❑ Agreeing to work the map at a high-level or in detail
❑ Maintaining focus on the current situation until the analyses have been completed
❑ Creating the map
❑ All types and stages of analysis
❑ Deciding what the new process could look like
❑ Agreeing how to progress implementation of changes
❑ Collecting data to check improvement has really occurred

Dealing with difficult moments

✓ Don't take it personally
✓ Focus on the facts and not the people or their values
✓ Clarify the question or issue
✓ Gather more information
✓ Slow down the debate; suggest time for reflection
✓ Listen actively
✓ Help others to participate
✓ Take turns to speak
✓ Respect and learn from different points of view
✓ Break large groups into pairs
✓ Connect on a personal level
✓ Ignore mildly negative behaviour and address very negative behaviour privately

Chapter 37

Different points of view

When asked what her biggest personal learning was in the mapping exercise, Gillian replied that it was understanding that different points of view not only mattered, but were ok. She explained how the map itself brought many perspectives together and that for many people, the realisation of their role came as a bit of a surprise. She also found people were quick to criticise what others were doing, but always then defended what they were doing in delivering the patient process! For example, one of the consultants spent a lot of time arguing that what the map demonstrated happened in the medical records department, was wrong. Medical records team members tried to explain that was actually what happened.

Gillian told the workshop that she had learnt enough to know that there were different points of view and there was always something to learn from them. The trick, she found, was to check the facts and acknowledge the different opinions without judging which was right or wrong. If someone felt a certain way about something, well, that was how they felt – it was not a matter of it being a wrong way to feel. She explained she used to spend quite a lot of time outside the meetings making sure she understood people's opinions and helping them to see and accept others' different points of view.

Everyone has their own point of view about a subject, and that is absolutely fine. Where this gets difficult is when one person tries to force their point of view on others. When this happens:

❑ Remember to focus on the one point of view that unites everyone – the patient's!
❑ Acknowledge the different opinions without judging them; ask for more points of view, record these, and allow time for reflection
❑ Return to the original objectives of the mapping exercise and improvement project
❑ Check the discussion is still within the definition of the process you're mapping
❑ Gather more facts and information
❑ Spend time understanding why it is someone holds a specific point of view and is being forceful about it. They may have other reasons they haven't yet shared with you

Switching roles

One way to show that you respect and value different points of view, and to help others experience what different team members my be thinking and feeling, is to carry out a short exercise where each person takes on a different professional role. You can do this as a 3–5 minutes exercise on any topic that is proving contentious or difficult.

You can either do this as an exercise where people discus the issue in the new roles in pairs or as a whole group, or you could ask everyone to take on the new role and write some notes about how you think the other person may feel about the issue. The second option is best used when the group is new and feeling a little 'unsafe'.

Learning from others

Different opinions are valuable. There is no need to judge them or resolve them. People can be allowed to hold different views about what is going on, especially if they are still able to participate in the mapping process. One way to acknowledge these opinions, especially early on, is to take one or two as examples and work them through. Capture the issues and reflect them onto the map. What do you learn from this? Write it down so everyone can see.

Annotated bibliography

Dettmer HW, "Goldratt's theory of constraints; a systems approach to continuous improvement", ASQ Quality Press: Wisconsin, 1997
A comprehensive guide to the theory of constraints, including ways to facilitate change using the theory. Best for the more advanced improvement practitioner.

Galloway D, "Mapping work processes", ASQ Quality Press: Wisconsin, 1994
A non-healthcare specific workbook that takes you through the detail of mapping a process. Useful for those who want to know more about mapping techniques. Best for beginners, though others will also benefit.

Hammer M, "Beyond reengineering; how the process-centered organization is changing our work and our lives", Harper Collins: London, 1996
Descriptive reasoning on why processes are core to business. Not healthcare specific.

Langley GJ, Nolan KM, Nolan TW, Norman CL, Provost LP, "The Improvement Guide; a practical approach to organizational performance", Jossey-Bass: USA, 1996
A definitive guide to improving processes in organisations. Introduces and explains the improvement model which includes the Plan-Do-Study-Act cycle. It is suitable for both beginners and more experienced improvement leaders.

Smith S (Ed), "Solve that problem; readymade tools of continuous improvement", Kogan Page: London, 1997
Short and simple guide to many useful tools for identifying problems, gathering data, analysing problems, generating ideas, making decisions and planning for action. Highly recommended.

Thor CG, "Designing feedback; performance measures for continuous improvement", Crisp Publications; USA, 1998
Simple guide to the variety of ways feedback can be designed. Not healthcare specific.

Womack J & Jones D, Lean Thinking, Simon & Shuster: New York, 1996
Industry related descriptive accounts and explanations of lean principles in action. Not healthcare specific and the examples are orientated around production lines.